YOUR KNOWLEDGE HAS VALUE

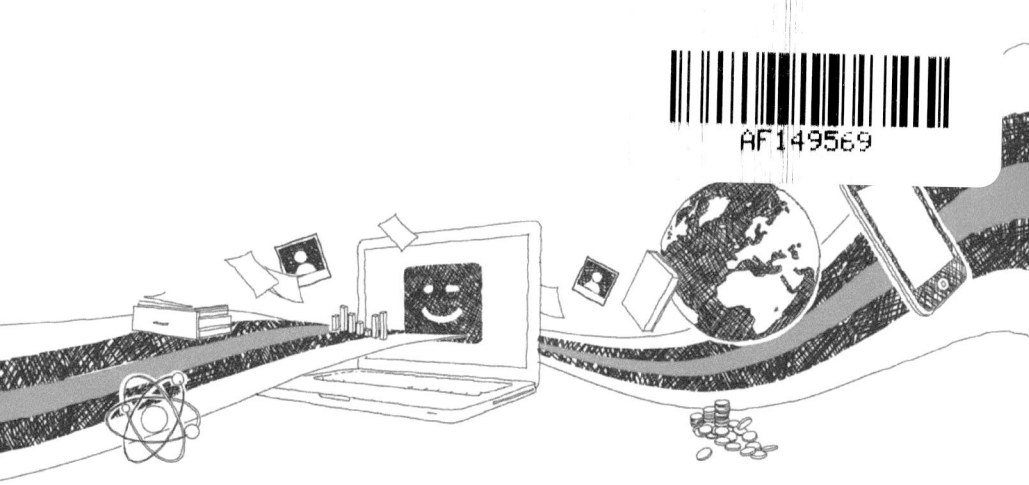

Bibliographic information published by the German National Library:

The German National Library lists this publication in the National Bibliography; detailed bibliographic data are available on the Internet at http://dnb.dnb.de .

Imprint:

Copyright © 2016 GRIN Verlag, Open Publishing GmbH
Print and binding: Books on Demand GmbH, Norderstedt Germany
ISBN: 978-3-668-24221-0

This book at GRIN:

http://www.grin.com/en/e-book/333865/information-systems-in-hospitals-and-the-health-service

Kamalesh Dey

Information Systems in hospitals and the health service

A critical report on "Increased electronic information sharing by sexual health services" by Hunter, Ede and Whiddett

GRIN Publishing

GRIN - Your knowledge has value

Since its foundation in 1998, GRIN has specialized in publishing academic texts by students, college teachers and other academics as e-book and printed book. The website www.grin.com is an ideal platform for presenting term papers, final papers, scientific essays, dissertations and specialist books.

UNIVERSITY OF BEDFORDSHIRE

MBA BUSINESS ADMINISTRATION

(HOSPITAL AND HEALTH SERVICES MANAGEMENT)

INFORMATION SYSTEMS IN THE HOSPITAL AND HEALTH SERVICES

MODULE UNIT CODE: SHR606-6

WRITTEN CRITIQUE REPORT

ON

HUNTER, HAINING EDE AND WHIDDETT'S (2014) ARTICLE

BY

KAMALESH CHANDRA DEY

08 MAY 2016

WORD COUNT: 2800

Content

Table of Contents   Page No

Introduction

The paper is a critique report of Hunter, Haining Ede and Whiddett (2014) regarding "Increased electronic information sharing by sexual health services: Confidentiality and consent" published in the health informatics journal. The purpose of this report is to appraise critically of Hunter, Haining Ede and Whiddett's (2014) article using CASP (Critical Appraisal Skills Programme) tool and comment with supportive evidence on the article by following standard review checklist (CASP, 2013). In addition, the article will be critically appraised through the various quality checklists (Quality checklist for the pilot study through questionnaire, Quality checklist for qualitative studies from Greenhalgh et al., 2008). Initially, the critique report will highlight on the author's published article. It will also explore the study aim, objective, study design, outcomes, and any encountered biases if any. Finally, the report will summarise the key points of the article in the light of significance of the information system in hospital and health service system and how the published article integrates to the information system with sexual health services in the hospital.

Critique report or Critical appraisal is the analytical process of full of attention and systematically investigating research to assess its reliability, and its significance and relevance with an individual context (Burls, 2009). In addition, While Chambers, Boath, and Rogers (2007, p.51) defined that "critical appraisal as the assessment of evidence by systematically reviewing its relevance, validity and results to specific situations". Moreover, in case of health research studies, critical appraisal is fundamental and significant component in term of evidence-based health services, treatment, medicine, and public health practice in the hospital or in the community what includes scrutinising the strengths, weaknesses, and the areas of improvement of a particular study (Fowkes and Fulton, 1991).

Hunter, Haining Ede and Whiddett (2014) presented in their published article regarding the implication of introducing the National Health Index (NHI) to share patient health information by sexual health services (SHS) with other external providers in New Zealand. This article, Authors inspected patient attitudes towards the modification in health services to support a combined model in the current care setting in New Zealand. Based on research outcomes, increasing sharing patient's information without consent among external health providers' would influence people to stop visiting in sexual clinic. Consequently, the rate of STIs could be increased, while currently STIs are very common in New Zealand even higher thank United Kingdom (The Environmental Institute of Science and Research, 2016). Therefore, the authors suggested that consent and confidentiality could be taken place in a serious manner in national health policy particularity for the patient in sexual health services.

Hunter, Haining Ede and Whiddett (2014) carried out significant research regarding sharing patient confidential information in sexual health services through UPI (Unique Patient Identifier) without patient's consent among various health services providers. Adler *et al.,* (2002) stated that sexual health is very crucial part of an individual in term of physical and mental health of an individual. It is an integral part of our identity as human beings along with important human rights to their privacy and dignity, social and family life, and living in the civil society with equal opportunities. Better sexual health is depends on some factors for instances good sexual relationship and adequate access to sexual health service centre what ultimately prevent the risk of STIs and unwanted pregnancy (Edwards and Coleman, 2004).

This article has been chosen to critique as its contextual significant regarding patient's confidentiality and sharing information without consent in sexual health services. Sexual health is very important issue for human being and STIs (Sexually Transmitted Infections like chlamydia, HIV) are the current global public health concerns. On the other hand, Patient confidentiality is also very important issue in term of sexual health service providers and obtaining consent would be necessary step before sharing patient's information to other health providers. Moreover, the critique will address the strengths and weaknesses of the published article based on supportive evidence and explanation.

Analysis

The following part of the report will analyse the article based appropriate evidence and logical explanation.

Authors highlighted that patient's health information sharing system is increasing among external health services providers electronically. Studied found that patients attending in sexual health service were unwilling to share their in health information. Therefore, it was major concern for the patients to attend the sexual health clinic. Consequently, rate of infection might be increased due to stop visiting sexual clinic. Author provided recommendation to Sexual health services as they could compromise their information sharing system based on patient's consent.

The authors conducted qualitative pilot study in local hospital based on Sexual health services in New Zealand. Data was collected through the distribution of questionnaire by the clinic receptionist to avoid any kind of biasness. Participants could complete the self-administered questionnaire into two ways for instances sitting in waiting areas or complete at home and send back by post in a prepaid envelop. However, authors did not mention their research question clearly based on PICO (Patient, Problem or Population, Intervention, Comparison, Control or Comparator, Outcomes) tools where they could identify the particular participants and specific questions in the questionnaire (Stolberg, Norman, and Trop, 2004).

In addition, the full article is evaluated through the numerous critical assessment criteria based on the Effective Public Health Practice Project (EPHPP) shown in the following table 1:

Table 1: Summary of the quality appraisal of the published selected article based the Effective Public Health Practice Project (EPHPP) (EPHPP, 2009)

Critique Assessment Criteria	Details
Study Title /Authors	"Increased electronic information sharing by sexual health services: Confidentiality and consent" / Hunter, Haining Ede and Whiddett (2014)
Aim & Objectives of the study	➢ To examine the patient awareness of NHI number and motive for clinic visits in SHS; ➢ To establish patient behaviour and attitudes to adopt NHI numbers in various health services for instances lab test result, discharge form, clinic visit history, ➢ To define possible negative consequences of sharing information to external service providers by SHS.
Study Time Frame	10 August to 11 September 2009
Study Design	Qualitative pilot study
Sample Size	Total 249 patients attended the Sexual Health Services
Ethical Considerations	Ethical approval was approved by the Central Regional Health and Disability Ethics in New Zealand
Definition Of Outcome Measure	A sequence of chi-square tests were used in the study to determine the patients' attitudes towards sharing their information to external service providers
Data Collection	Data was collected through the distributed on questionnaires
Data Analysis	Data was analysed along with the descriptive statistics and chi-

	squared tests through the PASW Statistics v18 software
Result	➢ 70% patient were unknown, 20% were known a little and only 10% were well known about NHI; ➢ In addition, findings suggested that female patients were more well-known compared to male patients ➢ Findings also recommended that patients were unwilling to share the information even their attendance in the clinic might be reduced
Limitation	There was maximum margin of error of ±6.9 per cent in the analysed results. In addition, NHI was not well known to all patients; therefore, patient response could be influenced through the better understanding about NHI.
Bias	Lack of patients awareness regarding NHI, result was more likely biased significantly
Quality Grade	moderate

Based on various appraisal tools, there are some strengths and weakness of the published article which are pointed in the following section:

Strengths
There are many strengths of the article which is discussed below:

The title is the most important element to evaluate instantly the quality of any article. The key words like sexual health service, patient confidentiality, and consent are the most important issue in the health industry. Therefore, the article title is quite durable and realistic (Crombie, 2011). In addition, abstract is also very crucial to evaluate the quality of the article. Bowling and Ebrahim (2005) stated that abstract gives the overview about the whole study as well as the research outcomes. As a whole, the article has met the criteria and this is the strength point of the article.

Regarding study aim and objectives, the authors tried to explore the patient awareness about the NHI number and actual motive of their clinic visit in the sexual health services. The authors also tried to fix up the patient behaviour and attitude to make familiarise with HNI number in term of various health service centre from primary to tertiary care level. Furthermore, the authors tried to convince to the health policy maker to redesign the electronic sharing information without patient consent and highlight the negative impact (stop visiting sexual clinic what might increase the risk of STIs) of sharing information especially in sexual health clinic data towards external health providers (Fernando and

Clutterbuck, 2008). The authors had clear and specific realistic aim and objectives in their pilot study what makes strong point in the published article (Moher et al., 2010).

EPHPP (2009) stated that project or research timeline is very important to produce a good quality research. Study was carried out from 10 August to 11 September 2009 what provided specific period of time. The authors conducted qualitative pilot study and used questionnaire to collect data from the patients. The questionnaire was collected from previous study of Whiddett et al. (2006) and designed to complete around 10 minutes. All participants were eligible if they were 16 years or over and had no mental problems or language barrier. In the pilot study, total 249 patients participated and filled out the questionnaire in the Sexual Health Services centre, while questionnaire was distributed by the receptionist to avoid any kind of biasness. In addition, participants would complete the questionnaire either in waiting room or at home and return the completion questionnaire by post in prepaid envelop. Consent was asked just before choosing participants. In addition, questionnaire and NHI number was also explained in the information leaflet to avoid any kind of confusion or dilemma (Hunter, Haining Ede and Whiddett, 2014).

Data was analysed through the descriptive statistics and chi-squared tests was done by using PASW Statistics v18 software, while highest margin of error of ±6.9% was found in the final result. Among 249, only 87% (216) participants completed the questionnaire. However, 209 respondents completed full questionnaire and 7 questionnaires were rejected due to incomplete information, where 80 (38%) were men and 129 (62%) were women respondents and overall the response rate was 84% in the study and 91% respondents were identified as heterosexual. The authors analysed properly the participant's feedback and discarded some questionnaire based on their completeness what was actually strong point and made quality research (Greenhalgh et al., 2008) (CASP, 2013).

In term of ethical consideration, the authors received ethical approval from the Central Regional Health and Disability Ethics in New Zealand. This is actually crucial consideration to conduct a good research (EPHPP, 2009). The authors completed this important part before data collection. This is also strong evidence of the article (CASP, 2013)

About 70% patients were unknown, 20% were known a little and only 10% were well known about NHI. In addition, findings suggested that female patients were more well-known compared to male patients. However, there was no relationship between well known and unknown about NHI. Therefore, there was a least possibility to produce bias result. The authors provided full explanation about biasness. These criteria act as strength of the research (CASP, 2013). In addition, the authors added the key findings of their study in the result section regarding NHI awareness and reasons for clinic attendance. The authors found some of the respondents (39%, 37% and 33%) were under may be group, however, most of the patients were unwilling to share their information (Hunter, Haining Ede and Whiddett, 2014).

Likewise, Whiddett et al. (2006) found same result in their previous study regarding patient sharing information. However, the maybe group were willing in some extent to share their personal information but they wanted to know more details before disclosing their information during hospital access, NHI use, discharge letter, and among other medical staffs. The authors designed questionnaire in such a way where participants could give their additional comments regarding increasing information sharing system by SHS and 20 patients gave their comments on that and mentioned as they need formal discussion and consent before sharing any types of health information. Moreover, patient's attitude towards sharing information was justified through chi-square tests. The authors found that only 16 to 19 years age group was statistically significant ($p < 0.05$) and disagree to disclose their sexual health information as well as deny to provide the history of clinic visits (Hunter, Haining Ede and Whiddett, 2014).

Moreover, the authors found some more findings regarding confidentiality and privacy based on text comments from participants. Most of the participants claimed that confidentiality ought to be maintained regarding sexual health sharing with other medical staff like their own GP. Majority of the participants disagreed to increase the system of sharing information; however health policy maker tried to extend their health service communication through the increasing sharing information electronically between GP and other external health services. However, the authors found both positive and negative consequences in term of clinic attendance due to increasing sharing information with or without obtaining patients consent. Majority of patients mentioned as they would be happy to revisit the sexual clinic again, while 62 out of 207 participants argued that they never visit sexual clinic even they would influence other people to stop coming to sexual clinic if NHI is shared with others (Hunter, Haining Ede and Whiddett, 2014). The final findings suggested that if SHS could really start increasing the sharing information system then patients could stop coming to sexual clinic. Likewise, Fernando and Clutterbuck (2008) found same findings in their study regarding clinic visit. They would be out of diagnosis and treatment of STIs. Therefore, the risk of STIs might be increased in the country (Whiddett et al., 2005).

Weaknesses
There are numerous strengths of the article what has been discussed in the earlier section. However, there are some notable limitations as well what is outlined below:

The study was dealing with the significant concerns along with new approach in health information system in New Zealand; however it was not fully successful and able to address the research question. The authors claimed that they will make awareness about NHI number but did not take any initiatives for instances introducing new programs or campaigns during the study. During data collection, questionnaire was not fully understandable due to NHI number as almost majority of the participants were unaware about NHI number. Well-known about NHI numbers, participants would be responded widely and effectively. Therefore, data might not be able to collect accurately or fluctuate minimally (CASP, 2013).

In addition, participants were only specific ethnic group like Maori and teenager but other ethnic groups like Asian and African people were not included in the study what could be the weakness of the study. Data was collected only from some general source of ethnic group what made the result in general instead of realistic and effective. It is essential to collect data from numerous sources to produce high quality research outcomes (Greenhalgh et al., 2008).

Moreover, the authors did just mention about ethical approval, while did not explain any more details about the process of getting ethical approval and how they applied through getting approval from the national health services in New Zealand. In term of good quality research, need full explanation of ethical approval (CASP, 2013). Furthermore, study was conducted in the rural outreach clinics in the large geographical region with a massive population. So, privacy and confidentiality might be varied in smaller areas like other parts in New Zealand. Therefore, the result might not be generalised for the whole country.

Conclusions

Privacy and confidentiality is the significant concern in sexual health service centre in anywhere in the world. The article dealt with the case where new electronic information system was introduced to share patient confidential information through UPIs (NHI) without patients consent towards external health service providers in New Zealand. There is huge debate going on among patient in SHS due to increasing electronic sharing their confidential information. Consequently, the patients are actually worried as their personal informational regarding SHS is sharing with numerous external health service providers without any kind of their consent. Findings suggested that patients would stop visit SHS and influence others as well not to visit SHS. Therefore, the attendance would be reduced and STIs might be increased due to increasing electronic sharing information to other health providers like GP, hospital staff.

The pilot project explored the patient's attitude and their behaviour toward sharing information. Therefore, government need to opt out sharing information system without consent to avoid reduction of the clinic attendance and increase awareness among patients about the NHI numbers and significant of sharing information system towards other health providers. However, it is mandatory to keep patient all information safe and confidential for all health services especially in SHS. Finally, this paper would be useful and supportive for health policy maker, health professionals and researcher to address the patients concern through negotiation with patients consent and maintaining their confidentiality in term of electronic information sharing system towards external health service providers.

Recommendations

There are some recommendations what might help to address the current concerns of the patients as well as increase awareness about NHI number.

Sexual health is very confidential areas in human being. Therefore, it is essential to maintain as much as possible. The study could improve their outcomes through initiating some of the pre steps like making awareness about NHI and UPIs along with explanation and its significant usage in the health services. Consequently, they might get better response in term of data collection and enough text comments about electronic information sharing system. The pilot study could extend their study period as well to make more response compare to the current outcomes.

Figure1: Decision making flowchart for sharing information

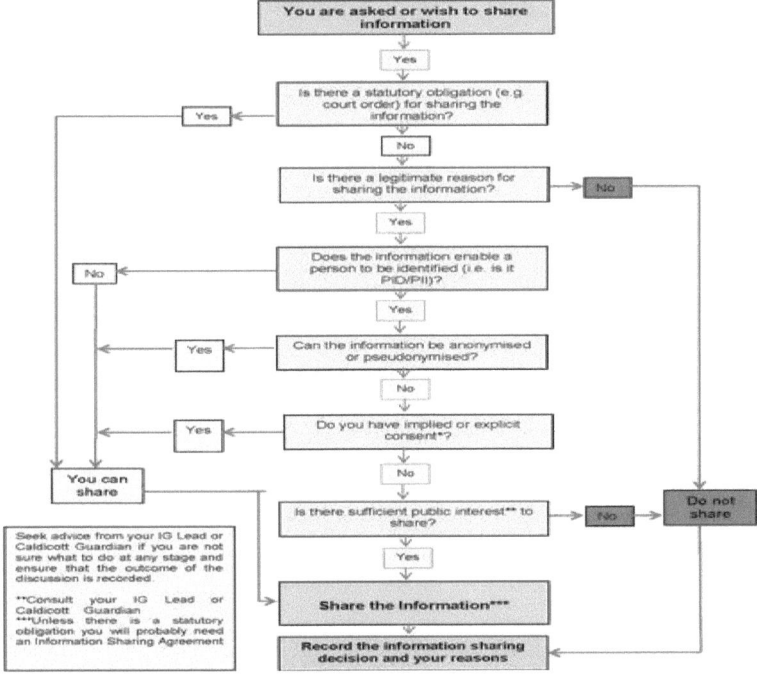

Source: South Staffordshire and Shropshire Healthcare NHS Foundation Trust (2013)

The health policy maker could implement new policy regarding increasing electronic information sharing system along with patient's consent (shown in figure 1). They followed the confidentiality law like as United Kingdom where not only sexual health service but also any patients information are kept in safe and confidential and consent is the pre requisite option just before sharing any kinds of information (South Staffordshire and Shropshire Healthcare NHS Foundation Trust, 2013).

Based on findings, patients could stop visit to sexual clinic due to electronic information sharing system. Therefore, STIs might be increased and that would be negative impact of the sharing information system. Before implementing the electronic information sharing system policy, government need to make aware the patients and let them know about the benefits unless it will not be effective policy and bring harm rather than getting benefits.

In addition, the government would initiate some new program where public patients could be aware about NHI and the new policy regarding electronic information sharing system towards external health service providers. Program could be related to discuss about the significant of NHI and the benefits of sharing information like to extend the patients communication with GP, local hospital as well as other medical staffs. If finally not work then government need to compromise their policy and add consent option where necessary for the patients to share their confidential information (Bratan, Stramer and Greenhalgh, 2010).

References

Adler, M.W., French, P., McNab, A., Smith, C. and Wellsteed, S. (2002) 'the national strategy for sexual health and HIV: implications for genitourinary medicine', *Sexually Transmitted Infections,* 78 (2), pp.83-86.

Bowling, A. and Ebrahim, S. *Handbook of health research methods: Investigation, measurement and analysis* Maidenhead, England; Open University Press, 2005.

Bratan, T., Stramer, K. and Greenhalgh, T. (2010) ''Never heard of it'–Understanding the public's lack of awareness of a new electronic patient record', *Health Expectations,* 13 (4), pp.379-391 [online]. Available at: http://onlinelibrary.wiley.com/doi/10.1111/j.1369-7625.2010.00608.x/pdf (Accessed: 02 May 2016).

Burls, A. (2009) *What is critical appraisal?* Second edn. United Kingdom: Hayward Medical Communications.

Chambers, R., Boath, E. and Rogers, D. (2007). *Clinical effectiveness and clinical governance made easy. Radcliffe Publishing Ltd* [Online]. Available at: http://books.google.co.uk/books?hl=en&lr=&id=qMSDTd5EYd0C&oi=fnd&pg=PR5&dq=Chambers,+R.,+Boath,+E.+%26+Rogers,+D.+%282007%29.+Clinical+effectiveness+and+clinical+governance+made+easy.+Radcliffe+Publishing+Ltd.+&ots=qm1Smwx1xh&sig=HbhNV0hGvkh-UWY47pG3lODlOQQ#v=onepage&q&f=false (Accessed: 10 April 2016).

Critical Appraisal Skills Programme (CASP, 2013). *CASP checklist for the qualitative study (pilot project).* Available at: http://media.wix.com/ugd/dded87_29c5b002d99342f788c6ac670e49f274.pdf (Accessed: 11 April 2016).

Crombie, I. (2011) *a pocket guide to critical appraisal: A handbook for health care professionals.* 2nd edition. London: British Medical Journal publishing group.

Edwards, W.M. and Coleman, E. (2004) 'Defining sexual health: a descriptive overview', *Archives of Sexual Behavior,* 33 (3), pp.189-195 [online]. Available at: http://0-

search.ebscohost.com.brum.beds.ac.uk/login.aspx?direct=true&db=afh&AN=13391907&sit
e=eds-live&scope=site (Accessed: 01 May 2016).

Effective Public Health Practice Project (EPHPP, 2009) *Quality assessment tool for
quantitative studies dictionary*. Available at:
http://www.ephpp.ca/PDF/QADictionary_dec2009.pdf   (Accessed: 27 April 2016).

Fernando, I. and Clutterbuck, D. (2008) 'Genitourinary medicine clinic and general
practitioner contact: what do patients want?', *Sexually Transmitted Infections,* 84 (1), pp.67-
69.

Fernando, I. and Clutterbuck, D. (2008) 'Genitourinary medicine clinic and general
practitioner contact: what do patients want?', *Sexually Transmitted Infections,* 84 (1), pp.67-
69 [online]. Available at: http://0-
search.ebscohost.com.brum.beds.ac.uk/login.aspx?direct=true&db=afh&AN=29365658&sit
e=eds-live&scope=site (Accessed: 20 April 2016).

Fowkes, F.G. and Fulton, P.M. (1991) 'Critical appraisal of published research: Introductory
guidelines', *BMJ (Clinical Research Ed.),* 302 (6785), pp.1136-1140 [Online]. Available at:
http://www.ncbi.nlm.nih.gov/pmc/articles/PMC1669795/?page=1 (Accessed: 16 April
2016).

Greenhalgh, T., Robert, G., Bate, P., Macfarlane, F. and Kyriakidou, O. (2008) *Diffusion of
innovations in health service organisations: a systematic literature review.* Second edn.
United Kingdom: John Wiley and Sons.

Hunter, I., Haining Ede, G. and Whiddett, R. (2014) 'Increased electronic information sharing
by sexual health services: confidentiality and consent', *Health Informatics Journal,* 20 (1),
pp.3-12 [online]. Available at: http://jhi.sagepub.com/content/20/1/3.full.pdf (Accessed: 20
April 2016).

Moher, D., Hopewell, S., Schulz, K.F., Montori, V., Gøtzsche, P.C., Devereaux, P., Elbourne,
D., Egger, M. and Altman, D.G. (2010) 'CONSORT 2010 explanation and elaboration:
Updated guidelines for reporting parallel group randomised trials', *Journal of Clinical*

Epidemiology, 63 (8), pp.e1-e37 [Online]. Available at:
http://www.ncbi.nlm.nih.gov/pubmed/20346624 (Accessed: 15 April 2016).

South Staffordshire and Shropshire Healthcare NHS Foundation Trust (2013) *Decision making flowchart for sharing information.* Available at:
http://www.sssft.nhs.uk/about/information-sharing-agreements (Accessed: 01 May 2016).

Stolberg, H.O., Norman, G. and Trop, I. (2004) 'Randomized controlled trials', *American Journal of Roentgenology,* 183 (6), pp.1539-1544

The Environmental Institute of Science and Research (ESR) (2016) *Sexually transmitted infections in New Zealand: annual surveillance report 2014.* Available at:
https://surv.esr.cri.nz/PDF_surveillance/STISurvRpt/2014/FINAL2014AnnualSTIReport.pdf
(Accessed: 01 May 2016).

Whiddett, R., Hunter, I., Engelbrecht, J. and Handy, J. (2005) "The Impact of Identifiability on Patients' Attitudes towards Sharing Their Health Information", *National Health Informatics Conference,* Health Informatics Society of Australia.

Whiddett, R., Hunter, I., Engelbrecht, J. and Handy, J. (2006) 'Patients' attitudes towards sharing their health information', *International Journal of Medical Informatics,* 75 (7), pp.530-541 [online]. Available at: http://www.ijmijournal.com/article/S1386-5056(05)00173-5/pdf (Accessed: 01 May 2016).

Bibliography

Fairley, C.K., Vodstrcil, L.A., Huffam, S., Cummings, R., Chen, M.Y., Sze, J.K., Fehler, G., Bradshaw, C.S., Schmidt, T. and Berzins, K. (2013) 'Evaluation of Electronic Medical Record (EMR) at large urban primary care sexual health centre', *PloS One,* 8 (4) [online]. Available at: http://0-search.ebscohost.com.brum.beds.ac.uk/login.aspx?direct=true&db=afh&AN=87677600&site=eds-live&scope=site (Accessed; 29 April 2016).

Johnstone, C. and McCartney, G. (2010) 'A patient survey assessing the awareness and acceptability of the emergency care summary and its consent model in Scotland', *Perspectives in Health Information Management / AHIMA, American Health Information Management Association,* 7 [online]. Available at: http://www.ncbi.nlm.nih.gov/pmc/articles/PMC2889371/pdf/phim0007-0001e.pdf (Accessed: 29 April 2016).

Maiorana, A., Steward, W.T., Koester, K.A., Pearson, C., Shade, S.B., Chakravarty, D. and Myers, J.J. (2012) 'Trust, confidentiality, and the acceptability of sharing HIV-related patient data: lessons learned from a mixed methods study about Health Information Exchanges', *Implementation Science,* 7 (1) [online]. Available at: http://0-search.ebscohost.com.brum.beds.ac.uk/login.aspx?direct=true&db=afh&AN=80127012&site=eds-live&scope=site (Accessed: 02 May 2016) .

Powell, J., Fitton, R. and Fitton, C. (2006) 'Sharing electronic health records: the patient view', *Journal of Innovation in Health Informatics,* 14 (1), pp.55-57 [online]. Available at: http://hijournal.bcs.org/index.php/jhi/article/view/614/626 (Accessed: 02 May 2016) .

Ward, R. (2013) 'Literature Review: The application of technology acceptance and diffusion of innovation models in healthcare informatics', *Health Policy and Technology,* 2 (4), pp.222-228.

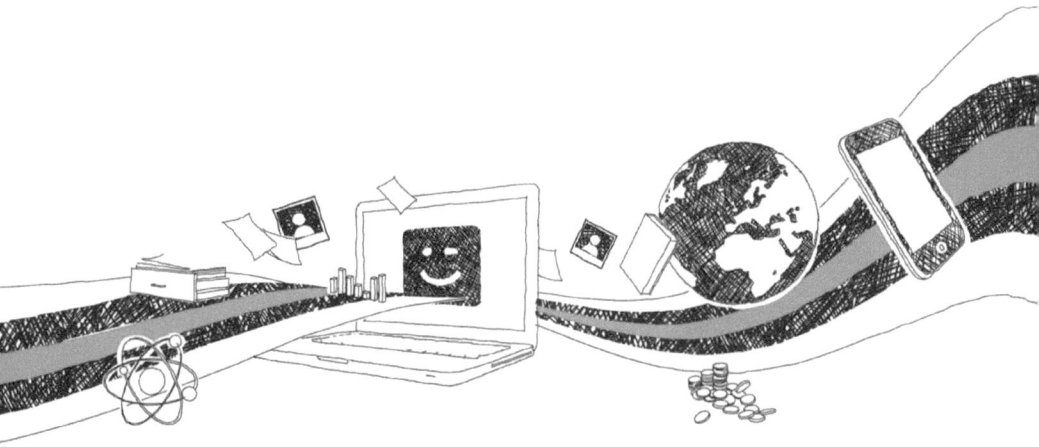
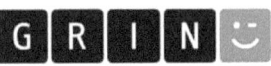